Discover remedies to heal back pain,prevent injuries,reduce anxiety,reshape your body with simple workouts and reclaim your life.

By

DR.joe waltern

This is an engaging book blurb on treating back and joint pain:

Introduction: Reclaim Your Power Over Your Life and Your Body

Are you sick of letting back and joint pain control everything you do?

Does your inability to do enjoyable activities stem from your stiffness and discomfort?

You're not by yourself.

These problems affect millions of individuals globally, yet there is hope.

This book is an all-in-one resource for comprehending and treating back and joint discomfort.

We'll examine common ailments including rheumatoid arthritis, sprains, and injuries as we investigate the underlying reasons of pain.

You'll find a variety of efficient treatment choices, including natural therapies, lifestyle changes, and conventional medical techniques.

This book gives you the tools to take a proactive role in your own recovery.

We'll cover techniques to reduce stress and inflammation, as well as useful exercises to increase strength and flexibility.

With clear explanations and practical guidance, you'll acquire the skills and information necessary to:

Determine the origin of your discomfort
Examine your alternatives for individualized treatment.

Adopt a holistic strategy for pain relief and healing.

Avoid relapses in the future and have a pain-free life

Give up on allowing back and joint pain to limit your life. Start down the path to long-term relief and an active, satisfying life.

This is a potent wrap-up for your book about curing joint and back pain:

In conclusion, embrace a journey of self-actualization and long-term health.

In this book, we have looked at how to treat joint and back discomfort.

You now know a great deal more about your body, available treatments, and your ability to control your pain.

Recall that healing is a process rather than a final goal.

Setbacks are inevitable, but with the knowledge and skills you've gained, you're suitably outfitted to traverse them.

Prioritize self-compassion as you proceed and acknowledge and appreciate all of your accomplishments, no matter how tiny.

Accept movement, pay attention to your body's cues, and don't be scared to get expert assistance when necessary.

Above all, give top priority to a way of living that enhances general well-being.

Eat healthily to fuel your body, learn how to handle stress, and adopt an optimistic outlook.

Recall that your suffering does not define you.

You are a resilient person who has the fortitude and wisdom to overcome obstacles and lead a happy life.

You may design a future free from pain and full of energy by adopting a holistic approach and taking responsibility for your health.

Table of contents

Chapter 1.

Understanding Leg, Lower Back, and Joint Pain: Regaining Control.

Hurt! Whether it's a sharp ache shooting down your leg after a long day or a lower back crick that makes getting out of bed seem like a Herculean task, we've all experienced it.

Millions of individuals worldwide suffer with leg discomfort, lower back pain, and joint pain.

These conditions are extremely frequent companions.

However, you don't have to accept that you will always be limited and in pain.

This chapter is the beginning of your journey to overcome pain and resume an active life.

We'll examine the causes of these frequent ailments, look into methods to locate their origin, and provide some insight on how to get you back on your feet (and pain-free!).

Recognizing the Cause of the Pain.

There are many possible causes of leg pain,lower back pain,and joint pain; some are mild and can be treated on their own, while others may call for medical attention from a specialist.

Below are a few of the typical suspects:

Frequent offenders include carrying heavy objects, hunching over our desks for extended periods of time, and repetitive actions like gardening that can lead to muscle tension or overuse.

Sciatica: The longest nerve in the body, the sciatic nerve travels from your lower back to your buttocks and down your leg.

This condition is caused by irritation of the sciatic nerve. Burning or severe shooting pain are possible side effects.

Chapter 2: Overcoming Muscle Soreness and Taming the Tightness.

Tightness and soreness in your muscles can ruin your day, much like unwanted guests at a party.

Muscle pain can seriously impair your pleasure of life, whether it's a dull ache after a weekend spent warrior-posing in the garden or a chronic knot that has been bothering you for weeks.

But do not be alarmed, fellow sufferer! This chapter serves as your manual for taking back control and getting rid of those bothersome aches.

The People Responsible for the Unease.

The basic causes of tense, cranky muscles are several. Presenting the typical suspects:

Overuse: Whether it's an extra set at the gym or a day spent bent over gardening, we've all experienced the sense of pushing ourselves a bit too far.

Inflammation and stiffness can result from small rips in muscle fibers caused by repetitive actions or extreme tension.

Posture: Although it may seem innocuous, slouching about all day puts uneven strain on your muscles, which over time can cause imbalances and tension.

Stress: It turns out that stress can have a disastrous effect on your muscles in addition to your head.

Your body releases tension hormones during times of stress, which causes your muscles to stiffen up.

Injury: Scar tissue from previous injuries, even those that appear to be mild, can limit muscle flexibility and movement, causing discomfort.

Get to Know the Foam Roller: Your Newfound Friend for Pain Relief

After identifying our adversaries, let's discuss some counterattack tools!

This is where the modest foam roller, your new best buddy, enters the picture.

This magical cylinder can be an effective tool in your toolbox for managing pain.

Self-Massage Techniques: You may help release those annoying adhesions and knots that cause tightness by gently pressing on your muscles and rolling them over a foam roller.

Imagine it as a deep tissue massage, except much less expensive and with far less awkward small conversation.

A fast internet search will teach you exactly how to target the individual muscle groups that cause your discomfort.

There are many different ways available.

Targeted Approach to Trigger Point Therapy.

Occasionally, the pain is localized, as if a small gremlin were squeezing a nerve.

Let's talk about trigger point therapy! These so-called "trigger points" are akin to extremely sensitive knots in your muscle fibers that have the ability to cause pain in other places.

Here's how to locate and turn them off:

Locating the Trigger Point: Examine your muscles gently to feel for any particularly sore areas.

Congratulations! You've found one when pressing on it produces a deep, aching feeling.

Your trigger point is there.

Applying Pressure: After you've identified the offender, press hard (without going overboard) on the trigger point for a half-minute or longer.

There may be some discomfort at first, but the pain should eventually go away.

Don't forget to maintain your muscular tone! Apply light to moderate pressure, and then release it if the soreness gets worse.

For best effects, try adding trigger point therapy and self-massage to your regimen a few times a week.

Consistency is the key in this situation.

Bonus Advice: Heat's Magic.

To improve the effectiveness of trigger point therapy or self-massage,apply heat beforehand to help relax the muscles.

Your muscles will benefit greatly from a warm compress or a brief dip in a hot bath.

You may take back control of your body and combat muscular soreness by implementing these tactics into your practice.

Remember that consistency is important !So grab your foam roller, inhale deeply, and bid those annoying aches a fond farewell!

Chapter 3.

Unleashing Your Inner Acrobat: Keeping Your Flexibility Throughout Life.

Do you recall how it felt to be able to bend into a pretzel as a child?

Back then, all of us were incredibly flexible, able to gracefully distort our bodies.

However, life throws us curve balls occasionally: extended periods of time spent hunched over desks,monotonous tasks, and the unavoidable passage of time.

Reaching for our toes feels, all of a sudden, like trying to high jump without ever getting off the ground.

Fear not, my fellow sufferers of stiffness! Being flexible isn't a forgotten art that only gymnasts and yogis possess.

Whatever our age or level of physical ability, it's an essential talent that we can all develop.

Good flexibility not only increases our range of motion, which makes daily chores like tying shoes or grocery shopping easier, but it also lowers our chance of injury and prevents bothersome back pain.

Consider it a miracle drug for an active, pain-free life.

How therefore do we find that thrill of movement again and kindle that inner acrobat within us? To get you started,here are some essential stretches.

The Hamstring Salute involves bending forward from the hips and reaching toward the ground while standing with your feet hip-width apart.

Allow gravity to lead you down instead of forcing it.

Bend your knees slightly until you feel a small tug, even if your hamstrings scream in protest (which they could!).

Breathe deeply, hold for 30 seconds, and then slowly roll back up.

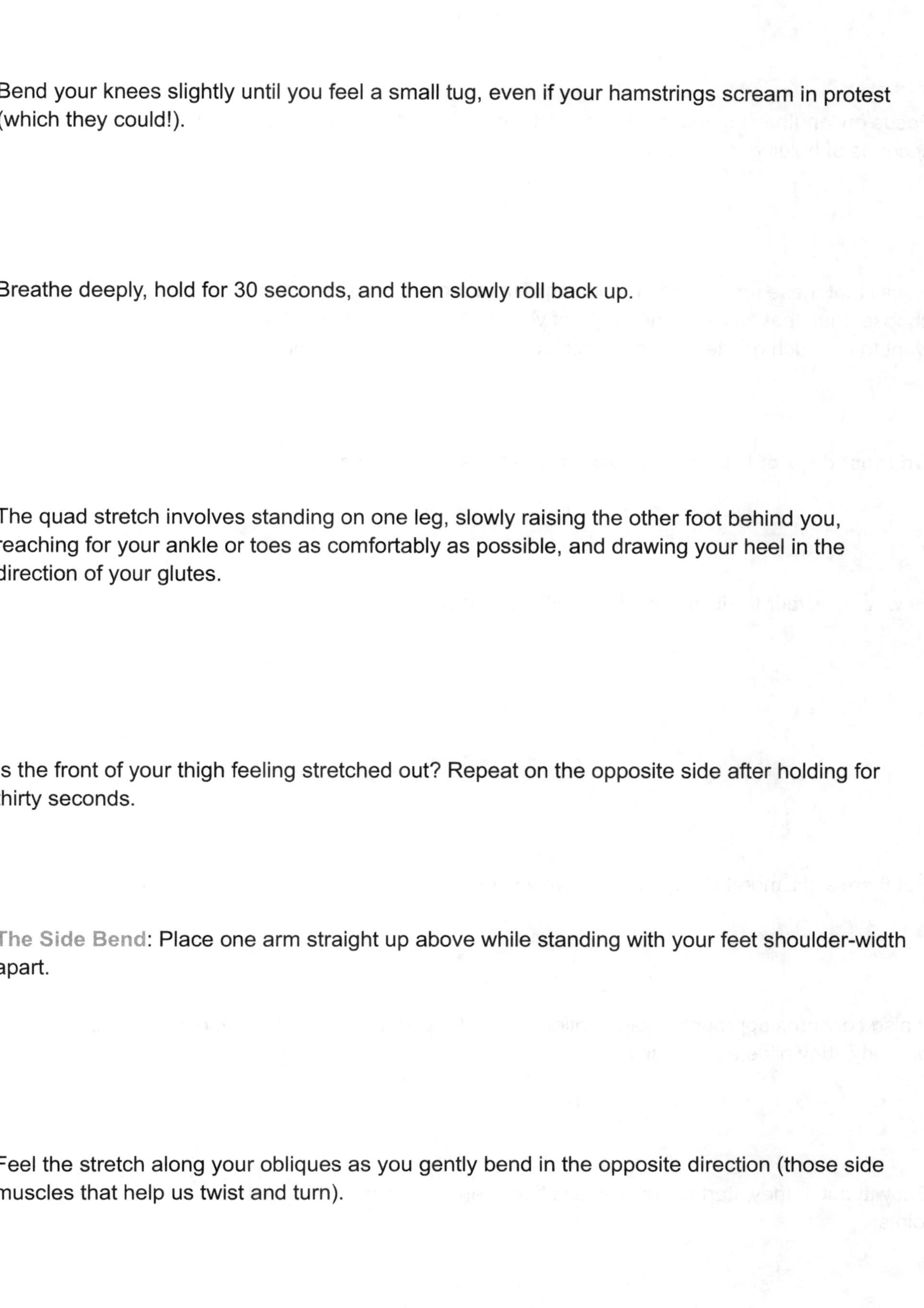

The quad stretch involves standing on one leg, slowly raising the other foot behind you, reaching for your ankle or toes as comfortably as possible, and drawing your heel in the direction of your glutes.

Is the front of your thigh feeling stretched out? Repeat on the opposite side after holding for thirty seconds.

The Side Bend: Place one arm straight up above while standing with your feet shoulder-width apart.

Feel the stretch along your obliques as you gently bend in the opposite direction (those side muscles that help us twist and turn).

Focus on lengthening your side body instead of worrying about reaching your toes. After 30 seconds of holding, swap sides.

Recall that these are only the beginning! There are many different types of stretches available; choose ones that focus on the areas of your body that are tight or that involve activities you want to do, such gentle yoga or dance courses. Consistency is important.

On most days of the week, try to stretch for a few minutes.

How rapidly your flexibility develops will astound you.

But there's still more! Being flexible involves more than simply your range of motion.

It also concerns appropriate joint motion. Consider your joints like door hinges; when they move properly, they glide effortlessly.

But without it, they start to crack and stiffen. Here are some tips to maintain the health of your joints:

: Make gentle forward and backward rotations of your shoulders, wrists, hips, ankles, and even your neck. To lighten things up, feel free to incorporate some humorous arm swings or leg kicks.

Cat-Cow Pose: This traditional yoga pose is very beneficial to the spine.

Beginning on your hands and knees, perform the cow posture by arching your back upwards while inhaling, and the cat poses by rounding your back and tucking your chin as you exhale.

A few times over, repeat this while paying attention to the soft movement of your spine.

The Moral of the Story: Consider flexibility as a self-gift.

It's a method of moving with confidence and ease, embracing life's adventures without being constrained by physical constraints.

Now spread out your mat, accept the discomfort of those initial stretches, and acknowledge each little accomplishment as your body rediscovers its amazing capacity for mobility.

You may always become your own personal contortionist, after all!

Chapter 4: Your Body's Superpower: The Healing Power of Rest and Repair.

It's true that suffering can be really annoying.

It disengages you from your favorite pursuits, interferes with your sleep, and makes you feel like a cranky troll stuck in a human body.

The good news is that your body has an incredible repair system that activates the instant you are hurt or overuse it; it is a master healer.

Consider your body as an advanced machinery.

Your body requires rest and repair times in order to operate at its best, much like an automobile needs time in the garage for maintenance.

This chapter delves further into the benefits of sleep, showing you how it supports your body's natural healing processes and makes you feel better.

The Strong Repair Team: Inside the Workshop of Your Body.

Envision a group of minuscule, industrious workers who are continuously monitoring your body, repairing tiny tears, and restoring compromised tissues.

That's precisely what occurs when you take a break, my friend.

Your body sends a full team of repair experts to work on the issue as you sleep and relax:

Inflammation Fighters: These men get to the scene of an injury quickly, much the way firefighters do when they put out a fire. They remove clutter and make a healing environment.

Consider cellular architects to be building workers.

Your diet's building blocks help them repair damaged tissues and make them stronger than before.

Blood Flow Boosters: These invisible runners give the wounded area the nutrition and oxygen it needs to heal.

: When Repose Turns Into Rejuvenation.

Sleep is important for your body's internal repair shop to go into overdrive; it's not just about getting some Zzz's.

Your body releases growth hormone when you are in a deep slumber, which is a super hormone that helps with muscle growth and tissue repair.

Additionally,it's a time when your brain absorbs information and integrates memories, which can greatly affect how much pain you perceive.

Here's some advice: Aim for seven to eight hours of good sleep every night.

Get a comfortable mattress, establish a calming sleep ritual, and give up using electronics before bed.

Your body's repair team is like a magic potion when you get a good night's sleep!

Beyond Sleep: There's No Need for Boredom During Rest.

Even while sleep is king, rest is more than just getting enough zzz's.

Here are some more strategies for giving your body the rest it needs:

Pain is your body's way of telling you, **"Enough is enough**." Pay attention to it.

Take a break from an activity if it causes you pain! Trying to push through can make the injury worse and take longer to heal.

Mindful Movements: Practices such as yoga, tai chi, and gentle stretching can enhance blood flow and induce relaxation, which can help with healing.

Magic of Meditation: By focusing on your breathing and stealing your thoughts for a little period of time each day, you can lower stress hormones, which can make pain worse.

The proper atmosphere is necessary for your body to heal, just as a plant requires sunshine and healthy soil to flourish.

Here are some pointers for setting up a healing sanctuary:

Reduce Stress: Healing may be hampered by long-term stress. To relax and soothe your body and mind, try deep breathing exercises or meditation.

Nourish Your Body: Eating a balanced, healthful diet gives your body the components it needs to cure itself. Consider lean protein, fruits, veggies, and whole foods.

Hydration Hero: Water is necessary to remove poisons and carry nutrients. Try to consume 8 glasses of water each day.

Recall that taking a break is a show of strength rather than weakness.

You may support your body's natural healing processes and create the foundation for an active,pain-free life by making rest a priority and providing your body with the resources it requires.

Chapter 5: Fighting Daily Anguish - The Guerrilla Strategies of Day-to-Day Living

Pain can be a genuine creep, let's face it. It appears out of the blue at the most inconvenient times,making a mundane task like getting groceries into a physical feat of flexibility.

But worry not, comrades in the fight against discomfort!

This chapter gives you the skills and information you need to become an expert in treating common pain.

The Common Suspects: Recognizing Causes of Pain.

Everyone has experienced it.

You stoop to tie your shoes when all of a sudden, your lower back gives you a sharp pain that makes you feel as though you had stubbed your toe (on a mountain!).

Oftentimes,routine actions that we take for granted are the root cause of these unexpected attacks.

Below are some typical offenders:

Slouching Superhero: While hunching over your phone or laptop may seem comfortable at first, it can negatively impact your posture over time and put undue strain on your neck and back muscles.

The Lifting Enigma: We frequently underestimate how much commonplace items weigh.

Lifting objects like laundry baskets, grocery bags, or even that mischievous child's toy incorrectly can cause torn muscles and backaches.

The Sitting Samurai: Prolonged sitting, particularly with bad posture, weakens your core and tenses your hip flexors, which can cause pain in your legs and lower back.

Taking Control of the Castle: Techniques for Managing Pain on a Daily Basis.

Now that you are aware of your opponent, let's prepare for combat! Here are a few easy-to-use yet efficient methods for dealing with common pain:

The Posture Patrol: Pay attention to your posture at all times during the day.

Maintain a straight posture with your shoulders back and shoulders relaxed, and align your ears with your shoulders.

Get an ergonomic chair for working at a desk and program reminders to stand up and move about every hour.

The Lieutenant Who Lifts: Don't slouch—squat! Bend at the knees when lifting anything, maintaining a straight back and a tight core.

Think of yourself as a powerful, robust weightlifter rather than a withering willow.

The Sitting Strategist: Get your blood flowing with a five-minute break every hour. Take a walk, perform some easy stretches, or just get up and reach for the ceiling. Your body will be appreciative!

Tools of the Trade: Arsenal of Pain Relief

Even with our best efforts, pain might still raise its ugly head from time to time. Here are a few more tools for your pain management toolbox:

Warriors of Heat and Ice: Heat treatment eases tense muscles, while ice treatment lowers inflammation.

For acute injuries, apply an ice pack; for muscle aches, use a heating pad.

Allies Over-the-Counter: Ibuprofen and acetaminophen are two over-the-counter medications that can help alleviate pain momentarily. However, before using any drug on a regular basis, speak with your doctor.

Supportive Gear: If you have lower back pain or hard lifting, think about using a lumbar support belt. Another important addition is arch support, which should be provided by a quality pair of shoes.

Recall: Avoid becoming dependent on painkillers.

These tactics are designed to give you the power to actively manage your discomfort rather than just suppress it.

You may transform daily tasks into pain-free successes by paying attention to how you move, including basic exercises, and using helpful tools.

Now take charge of your daily aches and pains and recover an active, pain-free life!

Chapter 6: An Anatomical Journey to Demystify Pain.

Ever shriek in astonishment after stubbing your toe?

It occurs so quickly—almost reflexively.

However, the yelp and the shooting agony are the outcome of an intriguing voyage taking place inside your body.

This chapter is an invitation to take a behind-the-scenes look at the amazing science that explains why humans experience pain.

See yourself as a detective assigned to solve the puzzle of pain.

The initial action? knowing the location of the crime.

Our bodies are complex networks of organs,tissues,and yes,even microscopic investigators known as nociceptors.

These specific nerve cells, which are dispersed throughout our muscles, joints, and skin, serve as our pain receptors.

Imagine for a moment that you bump your arm on a table corner by mistake.

Your skin's nociceptors are triggered by the hit, much like an alarm system.

These nociceptors, however, are more than just loud sirens.

Their signals move through your nerves like messages on a freeway, sending electrical shocks.

 The central nervous system hub is your spinal cord.

Here, the pain signal is transmitted to other neurons, some of which go directly to the thalamus, the brain's sensory relay center.

Consider the thalamus to be a large sorting office.

It picks up signals from sight, hearing, touch, and yes, even pain, throughout your body.

The pain signal is subsequently routed to other brain regions for additional processing.

The somatosensory cortex is one region that resembles a map of your body in the brain.

It assists you in determining the precise location of the discomfort,such as the throbbing sensation in your right elbow. But there's still more!

The limbic system is another region that resembles the emotional control center.

It incorporates an emotional overlay on top of the basic pain signal.

For this reason, stomping on your toe can cause emotional distress in addition to physical pain.

This complex dance between your emotional response and the physical signal determines how much pain you experience.

At last, information about pain reaches your brain's CEO, the prefrontal cortex.

It selects how to react after taking into account all the available data, including the location, intensity, and emotional response.

Shall you scream and remove your hand? Is it better to grit your teeth and endure it?

The intricate process by which pain emanates from a cut toe is an amazing feat of human anatomy.

By comprehending it, we can develop into more adept investigators, deciphering the signals our bodies provide us and choosing wisely how to handle discomfort and encourage recovery.

Therefore, keep in mind that a pang or an ache is more than just a coincidental feeling the next time you feel one.

You are living out a fascinating tale that is a monument to the amazing human body's creation.

Chapter 7: Turning Your Attention Away from Pain Management.

It's true that pain may be a jerk.

It throws off our schedules,robs us of our sleep, and can make even the most straightforward activities seem like climbing Mount Everest.

Our innate tendency is to defend ourselves,reach for the strongest analgesics, and grit our teeth through the ache.

But what if there's an alternative approach?

This chapter focuses on taking a step back and changing your perspective from treating pain to a more comprehensive healing strategy.

It's important to realize that pain is frequently a messenger—a body's way of telling you something needs to be done

. It's a signpost on your road to recovery as much as an opponent to be vanquished.

The Influence of Mentality.

Our minds are immensely strong.

They have the power to increase or lessen discomfort.

It seems as though the pain in our knee or the aching in our lower back are all-pervasive when we're fixated on them.

 But we can regain some control if we adopt a different viewpoint.

The following are some strategies to develop a pain-positive outlook:

Gratitude: Turn your attention to the areas of your body that are functioning well. Every day, set aside some time to acknowledge the resilience and strength of your body.

Acceptance: Give in to your suffering. Accept it, but don't let it define who you are.

Visualization: Picture yourself moving freely and with ease. Imagine yourself executing your favorite yoga posture or hiking without experiencing any pain.

Self-compassion: Treat oneself with kindness.

Don't give up if you don't notice results right away because healing takes time.

Reduce Stress,Increase Life.

Stress and chronic pain are like lousy roommates—they feed off each other. Our bodies stiffen up under stress, exacerbating existing pain.

And it's difficult to stay calm when we're hurt! So, it's crucial to disrupt this pattern. Here are a few methods for reducing stress:

Meditation: Even a short daily meditation session can significantly lower stress hormones and soothe the mind.

Breathe deeply: Inhale slowly and deeply from your abdomen. This easy method might trigger your body's relaxation response right away.

Practice mindfulness by being in the present.

Take in all that you can see, hear, and smell.

Don't think about the hurt or the future.

The Greatest Medicine Is Laughter: Discover the humor in daily life.

Spend time with the people you love and find funny.

Laughter is a very effective stress reliever.

Developing a Reparative Mindset.

Medication and physical therapy alone are not enough to promote healing.

It's about taking care of your spirit and intellect as well.

Discover interests and pastimes that you enjoy doing and that give you a sense of accomplishment.

Make sleep a priority, maintain a good diet, and stay in touch with your support network.

You may enable your body to repair itself from the inside out by surrounding yourself with healing energy.

Recall that this is a journey rather than a destination.

 Good days and bad days will come.

But you can reclaim your life and go beyond pain relief by adopting a holistic approach to recovery and concentrating on progress rather than perfection.

Chapter 8: Strengthening Your Body with Mobility Training Supported by Science.

It's true that living with chronic pain can leave you feeling stiff, creaky, and longing for days when things are easier.

But do not be alarmed, comrades fighting discomfort!

This chapter focuses on revealing the science-backed mobility training, the hidden weapon in your pain management toolbox.

Think of your body as a well-balanced orchestra.

You require every muscle, joint, and tendon to work in unison for your everyday movement symphony.

Discordant notes of pain are caused when a particular area of the performance becomes off-key due to tightness.

The conductor who leads each component to move with elegance and ease is mobility training.

The Significance of Mobility.

Consider mobility to be the basis of all movement. Wider ranges of mobility in your joints relieve strain on your muscles and lower your chance of injury.

Additionally, it enhances your balance, posture, and even coordination, which makes daily tasks seem easier.

The most enchanted aspect, though? With mobility training, you can move with greater freedom and enjoyment and pain can be greatly reduced.

The Stretch's Scientific Basis.

So how does science account for this phenomenon that relieves pain?

Enhancing joint mobility leads to improved brain-muscle communication,which is the main goal of mobility training.

The summary is as follows:

Enhanced blood flow occurs when you perform mobility exercises because blood is rushed to the affected areas, supplying vital nutrients for restoration and healing.

Improved lubrication: Mobility exercises help your joints glide more easily by releasing synovial fluid, which is their natural lubricant.

Decreased muscle activation: Your muscles won't have to work as hard to stabilize your movements as joint mobility increases, which relieves tension and pain.

Creating Your Own Mobility Schedule: It's All Up to You!.

Customization is what makes mobility training so wonderful.

You can customize it to match your unique demands and constraints,unlike a one-size-fits-all exercise program.

This is how to begin:

Determine Your Tight Spots: Take note of any places that hurt or feel stiff.

Is it your hamstrings that are always tight or your lower back that hurts?

After determining the offenders, concentrate your mobility exercises on those regions.

Remember, this isn't a contest for flexibility—start gently, go slowly! Start with mild stretches and motions,and spend at least 30 seconds in each pose.

Instead of intense agony, you should sense a tiny stretch. You can progressively up the intensity as your mobility gets better.

Pay Attention to Your Body: Mobility exercise is a dialogue, not a combat, with your body. If you feel pain, ease off and modify your motion.

Trying to ignore pain can make things worse.

Key to Mobility Training: The secret to effective mobility training is consistency.

Make time each day for mobility exercises, ideally as part of your warm-up or cool-down.

Aim for at least 10 to 15 minutes.

Mobility Activities to Win!

You can include a plethora of mobility exercises in your regimen, ranging from basic joint rotations to stretches influenced by yoga.

To get you going, consider these few examples:

Cat-Cow Pose: This traditional yoga pose enhances back mobility by strengthening and stretching your spine.

Foam rolling is a self-massage practice that enhances fascial mobility by breaking down tight muscle tissues.

Ankle Circles: Good hip and knee function depends on ankle mobility.

To extend the range of motion in your ankles, just rotate them in both directions.

Recall that your path for mobility is only getting started.

As you advance, try out several workouts to see which ones suit your body the best.

You can get more guidance from certified trainers and a wealth of internet resources.

You'll be well on your way to deconstructing the rusty machine and rediscovering the flexibility of pain-free movement by engaging in mobility training.

Recall that consistency is essential! Breathe deeply, move purposefully,and experience the delight of realizing your body's potential again.

Chapter 9: Customizing Your Corrective Exercise Program to Restore Your Body's Balance.

Pain, let's face it, can be a big downer.

It makes our regular routines more difficult, interferes with our workouts, and frustrates us.

We've discussed how to identify the cause of pain, overcome tense muscles, and even delved into the intriguing field of mobility training.

But what if your pain isn't just coming from tense muscles or restricted range of motion?

What if those twinges and tightness are the result of subtle or not-so-subtle imbalances that your body has developed?

Corrective exercises are useful here, my friend.

In the realm of fitness, they act as detectives, identifying any underlying postural abnormalities or movement dysfunctions that may be causing you discomfort.

Consider them customized adjustments to your workout regimen created to take into account the particulars of your physique.

I truly understand now what you might be thinking: "Personalized?

That seems difficult." But do not worry! The good news is that remedial activities are frequently surprisingly easy.

They don't need an Olympic-caliber training regimen or expensive equipment. Some of these movements may even be ones you're already familiar with from your regular workouts.

The secret is knowing how to adjust them to address particular imbalances.

Finding the Offender: Recognizing Unbalances.

So how might we recognize these disparities? These are some indicators that your body may be dropping:

Inconsistently slouching to one side: Do you notice this in your posture?

Does it appear as though one shoulder is always higher than the other?

These differences in posture may be a sign of abnormalities in your upper back or core muscles.

Pain during particular movements: Does a particular exercise routine consistently seem to cause pain in a specific location? This might indicate that a particular muscle group is overdoing it to make up for a poorer one.

Restricted range of motion: Do you find it difficult to bend deeply to one side or reach overhead?

This could be a sign of weakness or tightness in a particular muscle group.

See a physical therapist or a licensed trainer who can evaluate your movement patterns and posture if you observe any of these warning signs.

They can assist you in identifying particular imbalances and creating a customized exercise program for corrective action.

: Applying Corrective Exercises.

Let's look at a few instances now! Keep in mind that these are only suggestions; the particular exercises will change based on your own requirements.

Weak core, round shoulders: You can work on strengthening your core and challenging the stability of your shoulders by performing prone planks with alternating arm raises.

Hip flexors that are tight and limited in their elasticity can be stretched by performing glute bridges while raising just one leg.

Overcompensating on the dominant side: Single-leg workouts such as lunges and squats can help balance out muscle activation and improve the weaker side.

Putting Together Your Corrective Armory.

While you're creating your corrective workout regimen, keep the following important points in mind:

Begin slowly and advance step by step. Remind yourself that the goal of these workouts is to retrain your body, not to drive it to its limits.

Pay attention to form.

Prioritize quality before quantity! Correct execution of the exercises is more crucial than speeding through them.

Pay attention to your body.

Put a Stop to the workout and see a medical expert should incase you feel any pain.

Maintaining consistency is essential.

For best effects, try to work in corrective exercises two or three times a week.

You'll be positioning yourself for long-term success if you take the time to fix fundamental imbalances.

Corrective exercises aim to build a stronger,more resilient body that can move with confidence and ease rather than just treating discomfort.

Recall that your body is a wonderful mechanism that you can help realize its full potential and experience the joy of pain-free movement again with a little research and focused care.

Chapter 10: Strategies for Recovering from Injury: Get Back on Track.

Everybody has been there.

You stumble when playing that pickup game on the weekends, or perhaps you take on too much of that large-scale gardening project.

The world of agony suddenly becomes your unwanted friend.

Though it's a discouraging setback, do not be alarmed, fellow warrior! This chapter serves as your rallying cry and manual for getting back your life free of pain.

The Front Line of Protection: Repose, deference, and reevaluation
Following an injury, the early phases resemble a battlefield.

Your body yearns for sleep, much like a wounded soldier does.

Avoid pushing past the discomfort—it's an alert system signal.

Pay attention to it! While total inactivity is not necessary, it is important to move gently and give the damaged area time to heal.

Honor the Healing Process: It's Not a Sprint, It's a Marathon.

Although everyone wants their happiness right away, healing takes time. If the pace of progress seems slow, don't give up.

Consider it like building a house: you wouldn't anticipate a solid construction in a matter of hours.

Your greatest allies will be constancy and patience.

Reevaluating the harm: Talking to Your Medical Staff.

Certain injuries may heal on their own with proper care, but others may need to see a physiotherapist or doctor.

They are able to determine the full amount of the harm and suggest the best course of action.

Consider them your generals, planning the optimal response for your particular injury.

: A Balance Between Progress and Caution
When the first signs of inflammation go down, it's time to gradually resume movement.

Here, a physical therapist steps into the role of your drill sergeant, leading you through a customized fitness regimen. Take it gently at first, concentrating on stretches and workouts that won't make your injury worse.

Recall that the process is gradual and involves balancing prudence with advancement.

Developing Fortitude and Adaptability: Really, Scar Tissue Is Your Friend!
Scar tissue will form while you recuperate. Although it may sound unsettling, scar tissue is actually your body's means of mending damage.

It may, however, occasionally be constrictive and impede motion.

That's when targeted exercises and methods are useful.

You will develop strength and learn how to control scar tissue while working with your therapist.

Reducing Recurrences: Acquiring Knowledge from Your Errors
Accidents can provide insightful learning opportunities.

Consider what may have caused the injury. Was the form throughout the workout incorrect?

Did you undervalue how physically demanding a task was? Once you know the "why," you may take action to keep this from happening again.

Consider it as learning a new skill: the ability to move your body effectively and safely.

Remaining Upbeat: The Influence of Thought Over Matter
Sometimes the path to rehabilitation seems unattainable.

But keep in mind that an optimistic outlook is an effective tool in your toolbox. Concentrate on the little triumphs and acknowledge every advancement.

Techniques for visualization can also be beneficial.

Picture yourself regaining your strength and flexibility and moving without pain.

A positive mindset may greatly enhance the course of your recovery.

Recovering from an injury is a journey,not a destination, so keep that in mind.

You can quickly get back on the path to a pain-free life by adhering to these instructions,honoring your body's requirements,and maintaining your optimistic outlook.

Now, warrior, advance and triumph!

Chapter 11: Exercise Plans for a Life Without Pain.

Admittedly, the term "workout" may evoke visions of stomping, spandex-clad runners pounding the pavement or groaning weightlifters reaching their limits.

But worry not, my fellow sufferers! Though there may be joyous tears later, this chapter isn't about pushing oneself to the brink.

It all boils down to developing a movement regimen that works with you to live a pain-free life.

Consider your body as an exquisite, sophisticated machine.

You need to do routine maintenance on it to keep it operating smoothly.

Your body benefits from regular, deliberate movement rather than punishment, just as a car does not require continuous, high-octane racing.

The Enchantment of Low-Impact Activities.

Running or other high-impact exercises can be painful for your joints, particularly if you already have discomfort.

The good news is that there are a ton of low-impact activities available that can develop your body and improve your mood just as much.

Here are a few low-key celebrities to think about:

Swimming is a great full-body exercise that is easy on the joints and works your heart really well.

Walking is an easy, convenient, and highly beneficial exercise for increasing circulation, increasing stamina, and decluttering your mind.

Elliptical training: Without putting too much strain on your joints, this machine offers a low-impact aerobic workout that mimics running.

Pilates and yoga are examples of mind-body exercises that emphasize flexibility enhancement, core strengthening,and general wellbeing.

Utilizing bodyweight movements for strength training: Exercises like push-ups, planks, squats, and lunges are great ways to gain muscle without requiring expensive equipment.

Creating a Pain-Free Schedule.

Developing a training regimen that works for you means customizing it to your own requirements and tastes.

The following advice will help you get started:

Gradually build up the pace and intensity.

Don't expect to become a marathon runner overnight from a couch potato.

As you gain strength,progressively increase the duration and difficulty of your workouts from short, manageable ones to longer ones.

Pay attention to your body. Anguish is a warning, not a mark of pride.

Discover hobbies you love. It shouldn't be difficult to exercise.

Examine several pursuits and choose ones that you actually look forward to engaging in.

Change things up! Maintaining interest in your workouts and pushing various muscle areas requires variety.

Turn it into a gathering.

Joining a fitness class or going to the gym with a friend can provide accountability and fun to your workouts.

Sustaining an Active Way of Life for Long-Term Health.

The lovely secret is that even little amounts of activity throughout the day can have a big impact.

Instead of using the elevator, use the stairs, park further away and walk,stretch gently during the workday, or take a break to dance in your living room.

Every little bit matters!

Recall that consistency is essential.

You can live a pain-free life if you make regular, low-impact exercise a part of your schedule.

Not only will you feel energized and stronger, but however, you'll also be giving your body the freedom and delight to move.

Go forth now and take each pain-free stride toward conquering your day!

In conclusion, embrace a journey of self-actualization and long-term health.

In this book, we have looked at how to treat joint and back discomfort.

You now know a great deal more about your body, available treatments, and your ability to control your pain.

Recall that healing is a process rather than a final goal.

There will be obstacles along the way, but with the knowledge and skills you've gained, you'll be ready to overcome them.

Prioritize self-compassion as you proceed and acknowledge and appreciate all of your accomplishments, no matter how tiny.

Accept movement, pay attention to your body's cues, and don't be scared to get expert assistance when necessary.

Above all, give top priority to a way of living that enhances general well-being.

Consume wholesome nutrients to fuel your body, learn how to handle stress,Develop a positive outlook.

Recall that your suffering does not define you.

You are a resilient person who has the fortitude and wisdom to overcome obstacles and lead a happy life.

You may design a future free from pain and full of energy by adopting a holistic approach and taking responsibility for your health.